Osteoporosis Diet Cookbook for Women

Nourish Your Bones and Body With Calcium-rich Diet Recipes

Dr Olivia Tastewell

Copyright © 2024 by Dr Olivia Tastewell

Kindly scan the barcode below to reach out to the author and have access to more of our books.

TABLE OF CONTENTS

Introduction 6

Chapter 1: Breakfast Recipes 11

Panna Cotta with Blueberry, Prune Compote, and Cinnamon ..11

Skyr Yogurt Panna Cotta with Raspberries, Flax Seed, Peppermint, and Cocoa Powder 15

Citrus Berry Smoothie 17

Banana and Almond Smoothie 20

Oatmeal with Berries and Nuts 23

Chapter 2: Lunch Recipes 26

Vegetarian Pita..26

Turkey-Roquefort Salad...28

Spinach and Ricotta Cannelloni 31

Smoked Gouda Alaskan King Crab Mac 'n Cheese 34

Spinach Salad with Herbs, Goat Cheese, and Cashews 37

Chapter 3: Dinner Recipes 40

Veal Cordon Bleu 40

Lamb Tagine with Prunes, Almonds, Sesame Seeds, and Yogurt Sauce...42

Harri's Sardine Sandwich with Mustard & Yogurt Butter.........46

Spinach and Ricotta Parcels....................................48

Pumpkin and Kale Soup...51

Salmon and Broccoli Quiche 54

Chicken and Vegetable Curry 56

Greek Salad...58

Tofu and Vegetable Stir-Fry 61

Cheese and Tomato Pizza 64

Conclusion 67

Introduction

RACHAEL HAS ALWAYS BEEN A STRONG and active woman. She loved hiking, biking, gardening, and playing with her grandchildren. She never thought much about her bones, until the day she slipped on a wet floor and broke her wrist.

The doctor told her she had osteoporosis, a condition that causes the bones to become weak and brittle. He said it was common among women after menopause, and that it increased the risk of fractures and other health problems. He prescribed her some medication and advised her to eat more calcium-rich foods.

Rachael felt scared and confused. She wondered how she could prevent further bone loss and protect her health. She wondered what foods she should eat and what foods she should avoid. She wondered if she could still enjoy her favorite activities and hobbies. She decided to do some research and learn more about osteoporosis and nutrition.

She discovered that there was a lot of information and advice available, but not all of it was reliable or consistent. She also found that many of the recipes and meal plans she came across were boring, bland, or complicated. She wanted to eat well and keep her bones strong, but she also wanted to enjoy her food and her life. She wanted to eat foods that were delicious, satisfying, and easy to prepare. She wanted to eat foods that were good for her bones and her body.

That's why she created this cookbook for herself and other women like her. In this book, she shares 20 recipes for breakfast, lunch, and dinner that are specially designed for women with osteoporosis. These recipes are based on the latest scientific research and recommendations from experts in the field of nutrition and bone health. They are also inspired by her personal experience and preferences. She hopes that this cookbook will help you to nourish your bones and your body, by providing you with the nutrients you need, such as calcium, vitamin D, protein, and antioxidants. She also hopes that this cookbook will help you to enjoy your food and your life, by offering you a variety of foods that are tasty, filling, and simple to make.

She invites you to join her on this journey of discovery and delight. She invites you to learn more about osteoporosis and nutrition, and how they affect your health and well-being. She invites you to try some of the recipes in this book and to share them with your family and friends.

She invites you to eat well and keep your bones strong. Are you ready to accept her invitation? Are you ready to explore the world of food and flavor? Are you ready to nourish your bones and your body? If you are, then turn the page, and let's get started!

Chapter 1: Breakfast Recipes

Panna Cotta with Blueberry, Prune Compote, and Cinnamon

Ingredients:

- For the panna cotta:
    - 1 cup heavy cream (light cream or unsweetened almond milk alternative)
    - 1/4 cup whole milk
    - 1/4 cup granulated sugar
    - 1/2 teaspoon vanilla extract
    - 1/4 teaspoon unflavored gelatin powder
    - 2 tablespoons cold water
- For the prune compote:
    - 1/2 cup dried prunes, chopped
    - 1/4 cup water
    - 1 tablespoon lemon juice
    - 1 teaspoon honey
- For the topping:
    - 1/2 cup fresh blueberries
    - Ground cinnamon

Nutritional Information (per serving):

- Calories: 350 (based on using light cream)
- Fat: 20g (8g saturated)
- Carbs: 30g (4g fiber)
- Protein: 5g
- Calcium: 300mg (30% DV)

Cooking Time: 4 hours (chilling time)

Serving size: 2

Instructions:

1. Make the compote: In a small saucepan, combine prunes, water, lemon juice, and honey. Bring to a simmer and cook for 10 minutes, or until prunes are softened and compote thickens slightly. Set aside to cool.
2. Make the panna cotta: In a small bowl, sprinkle gelatin over cold water and let it bloom for 5 minutes.
3. In a saucepan, heat cream, milk, and sugar over medium heat until simmering. Remove from the heat and add the vanilla extract.

4. Whisk in the bloomed gelatin until dissolved.
5. Divide the mixture evenly between two ramekins or serving glasses. Cover with plastic wrap and refrigerate for at least 4 hours, or until set.
6. When ready to serve, top each panna cotta with blueberry compote and sprinkle with ground cinnamon.

Label: Creamy and light dessert, rich in calcium and antioxidants, customizable with different fruits and spices, and a good source of fiber.

Skyr Yogurt Panna Cotta with Raspberries, Flax Seed, Peppermint, and Cocoa Powder

Ingredients:

- 1/2 cup plain skyr yogurt
- 1/4 cup unsweetened almond milk
- 1 tablespoon honey
- 1/2 teaspoon vanilla extract
- 1/4 teaspoon unflavored gelatin powder
- 2 tablespoons cold water
- 1/4 cup fresh raspberries
- 1 teaspoon ground flax seeds
- Fresh mint leaves, for garnish (optional)
- Unsweetened cocoa powder, for dusting (optional)

Nutritional Information (per serving):

- Calories: 200
- Fat: 5g (1g saturated)
- Carbs: 20g (5g fiber)
- Protein: 15g
- Calcium: 350mg (35% DV)

Cooking Time: 4 hours (chilling time)

Serving Size: 1

Instructions:

1. Make the panna cotta: Follow steps 1-4 from the blueberry panna cotta recipe, using skyr yogurt instead of cream and milk.
2. Divide the mixture into two small ramekins or serving glasses. Cover with plastic wrap and refrigerate for at least 4 hours, or until set.
3. Prepare the topping: In a small bowl, mix raspberries with ground flax seeds and stir until coated. Allow 5 minutes to thicken somewhat.
4. When ready to serve, top each panna cotta with the raspberry mixture. Garnish with fresh mint leaves and a dusting of cocoa powder (optional).

Label: Protein-rich and high in calcium, vegan and gluten-free option, antioxidant-packed, refreshing, and light dessert.

Citrus Berry Smoothie

Ingredients:

- 1 cup plain yogurt (low-fat Greek yogurt recommended)
- 1/2 cup orange juice (freshly squeezed preferred)
- 1/4 cup frozen berries (mixed or your favorite type)
- 1/4 cup unsweetened almond milk
- 1/2 banana, frozen
- 1/2 teaspoon ground flax seeds
- Pinch of cinnamon

Nutritional Information (per serving):

- Calories: 300
- Fat: 5g (1g saturated)
- Carbs: 40g (5g fiber)
- Protein: 20g
- Calcium: 300mg (30% DV)

Cooking Time: 5 minutes

Serving Size: 1

Instructions:

1. In a blender, combine all of the ingredients and mix until smooth and creamy. Add more almond milk if necessary to adjust the consistency.
2. Pour into a glass and enjoy!

Label: Refreshing and nutrient-rich breakfast, a good source of protein, calcium, and vitamin C, vegan and gluten-free option, customizable with different fruits and spices.

Banana and Almond Smoothie

Ingredients:

- 1 frozen banana, chopped
- 1/2 cup plain yogurt (low-fat Greek yogurt recommended)
- 1/4 cup unsweetened almond milk
- 1 tablespoon almond butter
- 1/2 teaspoon honey (optional)
- 1/4 teaspoon ground cinnamon (optional)
- Pinch of nutmeg (optional)

Nutritional Information (per serving):

- Calories: 300
- Fat: 10g (2g saturated)
- Carbs: 40g (5g fiber)
- Protein: 15g
- Calcium: 300mg (30% DV)

Cooking Time: 5 minutes

Serving Size: 1

Instructions:

1. In a blender, combine all of the ingredients and mix until smooth and creamy. Add more almond milk if necessary to adjust the consistency.
2. Pour into a glass and enjoy!

Label: Creamy and satisfying smoothie, rich in potassium and healthy fats, high in protein and calcium, dairy-free option (use plant-based yogurt), vegan option (omit honey).

Oatmeal with Berries and Nuts

Ingredients:

- 1/2 cup rolled oats
- 1 cup water or milk (dairy or plant-based)
- 1/4 cup fresh berries (mixed or your favorite type)
- 1 tablespoon chopped nuts or seeds (walnuts, almonds, chia seeds, etc.)
- 1/4 teaspoon honey (optional)
- 1/4 teaspoon cinnamon (optional)
- Pinch of nutmeg (optional)

Nutritional Information (per serving):

- Calories: 300
- Fat: 10g (2g saturated)
- Carbs: 45g (7g fiber)
- Protein: 10g
- Calcium: 100mg (10% DV)

Cooking Time: 10 minutes

Serving Size: 1

Instructions:

1. Bring the water or milk to a boil in a saucepan. Stir in rolled oats and reduce heat to simmer. Cook for 5-7 minutes, or until oatmeal is thickened and creamy.
2. Remove from heat and stir in berries, nuts or seeds, honey (optional), cinnamon, and nutmeg (optional).
3. Serve warm and enjoy!

Label: Heart-healthy breakfast option, a good source of fiber and vitamin C, customizable with different toppings and spices, gluten-free option (use certified gluten-free oats).

Chapter 2: Lunch Recipes

Vegetarian Pita

Ingredients:

- 1 whole wheat pita bread
- 1/2 cup hummus (original or roasted red pepper flavor)
- 1/4 cup sliced cucumber
- 1/4 cup chopped tomato
- 1/4 cup crumbled feta cheese
- 1/4 cup mixed greens
- 1 tablespoon chopped fresh parsley
- Olive oil and lemon juice for drizzling (optional)

Nutritional Information (per serving):

- Calories: 350
- Fat: 10g (2g saturated)
- Carbs: 40g (5g fiber)
- Protein: 15g
- Calcium: 200mg (20% DV)

Cooking Time: 5 minutes

Serving Size: 1

Instructions:

1. Spread hummus evenly inside the pita bread.
2. Layer cucumber, tomato, feta cheese, and mixed greens.
3. Sprinkle with chopped parsley and drizzle with olive oil and lemon juice (optional).
4. Enjoy fresh and flavorful!

Label: High in fiber and plant-based protein, customizable with different vegetables and spreads, gluten-free and dairy-free options (use hummus without feta and choose a non-dairy cheese alternative).

Turkey-Roquefort Salad

Ingredients:

- 4 ounces mixed greens
- 3 ounces cooked sliced turkey breast
- 1/4 cup crumbled Roquefort cheese (or blue cheese alternative)
- 1/4 cup chopped walnuts
- 2 tablespoons apple cider vinegar or balsamic vinaigrette
- 1 tablespoon olive oil
- Salt and pepper to taste

Nutritional Information (per serving):

- Calories: 400
- Fat: 20g (4g saturated)
- Carbs: 10g (3g fiber)
- Protein: 35g
- Calcium: 150mg (15% DV)

Cooking Time: 10 minutes

Serving Size: 1

Instructions:

1. Toss mixed greens and turkey breast in a large bowl.
2. Sprinkle with crumbled Roquefort cheese and walnuts.
3. Whisk together vinegar or vinaigrette, olive oil, salt, and pepper.
4. Pour the dressing on the salad and mix it well.
5. Enjoy a protein-packed and flavorful salad!

Label: Rich in calcium and protein, bold flavor combination, gluten-free option (use gluten-free bread croutons if desired).

Spinach and Ricotta Cannelloni

Ingredients:

- 12 large lasagna noodles
- 15 ounces ricotta cheese
- 1/2 cup chopped spinach
- 1/4 cup grated Parmesan cheese
- 1/4 cup chopped fresh basil
- 1/4 cup marinara sauce
- 1 cup mozzarella cheese, shredded
- Olive oil for coating

Nutritional Information (per serving):

- Calories: 450
- Fat: 20g (8g saturated)
- Carbs: 40g (4g fiber)
- Protein: 30g
- Calcium: 400mg (40% DV)

Cooking Time: 30 minutes

Serving Size: 2

Instructions:

1. Preheat your oven to 375°F (190°C). Put a bit of olive oil on a baking dish.
2. Cook the lasagna noodles following the instructions until they're just right. Then, rinse them with cold water.
3. In a bowl, mix ricotta cheese, spinach, Parmesan cheese, and basil.
4. Spread a thin layer of marinara sauce on the bottom of the baking dish.
5. Fill each lasagna noodle with the ricotta mixture and roll them up. Put the rolled noodles with the seam down in the baking dish.
6. Pour the rest of the marinara sauce over the cannelloni, and add shredded mozzarella cheese on top.
7. Bake it for 20-25 minutes until the cheese is all melty and bubbly.
8. Let stand for 5 minutes before serving.

Label: Vegetarian comfort food option, rich in calcium and protein, customizable with different fillings and sauces, gluten-free option (use gluten-free lasagna noodles).

Smoked Gouda Alaskan King Crab Mac 'n Cheese

Ingredients:

- 12 ounces elbow macaroni
- 4 tablespoons unsalted butter
- 4 tablespoons all-purpose flour
- 4 cups whole milk
- 12 ounces smoked Gouda cheese, grated (plus extra for topping)
- 1/2 cup grated Parmesan cheese
- 1 tablespoon Dijon mustard
- 1/2 teaspoon paprika
- Salt and pepper to taste
- 8 ounces cooked Alaskan king crab meat, flaked

Nutritional Information (per serving):

- Calories: 550
- Fat: 30g (15g saturated)
- Carbs: 50g (5g fiber)
- Protein: 30g
- Calcium: 350mg (35% DV)

Cooking Time: 20 minutes

Serving Size: 4

Instructions:

1. Heat your oven to 375°F (190°C). Cook the macaroni as per the package instructions until it's just right, then drain it and set it aside.
2. In a big saucepan, melt some butter over medium heat. Stir in the flour and cook for about a minute.
3. Slowly mix in the milk, bringing it to a simmer. Keep whisking constantly until it thickens. Then, lower the heat.
4. Add smoked Gouda cheese, Parmesan cheese, Dijon mustard, and paprika. Season with salt and pepper to taste. Stir until the cheese is melted and the sauce is smooth.
5. Fold in cooked macaroni and crab meat.
6. Transfer the macaroni mixture to a baking dish and sprinkle with additional smoked Gouda cheese.
7. Bake for 15-20 minutes or until bubbly and golden brown.

8. Enjoy a decadent and protein-rich mac 'n cheese!

Label: Creamy and flavorful comfort food, a good source of calcium and protein, customizable with different cheeses and seafood (shrimp, lobster), gluten-free option (use gluten-free pasta).

Spinach Salad with Herbs, Goat Cheese, and Cashews

Ingredients:

- 4 cups baby spinach
- 1/2 cup crumbled goat cheese
- 1/4 cup sliced red onion
- 1/4 cup chopped dried cranberries
- 1/4 cup roasted cashews
- 2 tablespoons olive oil
- 2 tablespoons apple cider vinegar
- 1 teaspoon honey
- 1/2 teaspoon Dijon mustard
- Salt and pepper to taste

Nutritional Information (per serving):

- Calories: 300
- Fat: 15g (3g saturated)
- Carbs: 20g (3g fiber)
- Protein: 10g
- Calcium: 100mg (10% DV)

Cooking Time: 10 minutes

Serving Size: 2

Instructions:

1. In a large bowl, toss together spinach, red onion, dried cranberries, and cashews.
2. In a small jar, combine olive oil, apple cider vinegar, honey, and Dijon mustard. Shake well to emulsify.
3. Drizzle the dressing over the salad and toss to coat.
4. Crumble goat cheese over the salad and enjoy a fresh and flavorful lunch!

Label: Refreshing and light salad, rich in antioxidants and vitamins, vegetarian and gluten-free option (use vegan cheese alternative), customizable with different greens, fruits, and nuts.

Chapter 3: Dinner Recipes

Veal Cordon Bleu

Ingredients:

- 4 veal cutlets (4-5 oz each, pounded thin)
- 4 slices ham (thinly sliced)
- 4 slices Swiss cheese (thinly sliced)
- 1/2 cup all-purpose flour
- 2 large eggs, beaten
- 1 cup panko breadcrumbs
- 2 tablespoons olive oil
- Salt and pepper to taste
- Optional: lemon wedges and parsley sprigs for garnish

Nutritional Information (per serving):

- Calories: 450
- Fat: 25g (7g saturated)
- Carbs: 35g (2g fiber)
- Protein: 40g
- Calcium: 200mg (20% DV)

Cooking Time: 30 minutes

Serving Size:

Instructions:

1. Place each veal cutlet between two pieces of plastic wrap and pound thin with a meat mallet.
2. Season both sides with salt and pepper.
3. Place a slice of ham and cheese on each cutlet. Roll the item tightly and use toothpicks to hold it together.
4. Set up three shallow dishes for dredging: flour, beaten eggs, and panko breadcrumbs.
5. Coat each rolled cutlet in flour, then dip in egg, and finally coat generously with breadcrumbs.
6. Warm up olive oil in a big frying pan on medium heat. Add veal rolls and cook for 3-4 minutes per side or until golden brown and cooked through.
7. Take it off the heat and allow it to sit for 5 minutes before serving. Garnish with lemon wedges and parsley sprigs (optional).

Label: Rich and flavorful dish, customizable with different cheeses and meats, a good source of protein, gluten-free option (use gluten-free breadcrumbs).

Lamb Tagine with Prunes, Almonds, Sesame Seeds, and Yogurt Sauce

Ingredients:

- 1 pound boneless lamb shoulder, cut into bite-sized pieces
- 1 tablespoon olive oil
- 1 onion, chopped
- 2 cloves garlic, minced
- 1 teaspoon ground ginger
- 1/2 teaspoon turmeric
- 1/4 teaspoon cinnamon
- 1/4 teaspoon cayenne pepper (optional)
- 1 (14.5 oz) can of diced tomatoes, undrained
- 1/2 cup chicken broth
- 1/4 cup dried prunes, chopped
- 1/4 cup sliced almonds
- 1 tablespoon sesame seeds
- 1/2 cup plain yogurt
- Salt and pepper to taste
- Couscous or another grain, for serving

Nutritional Information (per serving):

- Calories: 400
- Fat: 15g (3g saturated)
- Carbs: 40g (5g fiber)
- Protein: 35g
- Calcium: 300mg (30% DV)

Cooking Time: 1 hour 30 minutes

Serving Size: 4

Instructions:

1. Heat olive oil in a large Dutch oven or tagine over medium heat. Brown lamb pieces on all sides.
2. Add onion, garlic, ginger, turmeric, cinnamon, and cayenne pepper (optional). Cook for 5 minutes, until fragrant.
3. Stir in tomatoes, chicken broth, prunes, and almonds. Season with salt and pepper.
4. Bring to a simmer, cover, and cook for 1 hour, or until lamb is tender.
5. Stir in sesame seeds and yogurt during the last 10 minutes of cooking.

6. Serve lamb tagine over couscous or another
    grain, spooning sauce over the top.

Label: Warm and comforting dish, rich in vitamin D
and calcium, gluten-free option (served with rice
instead of couscous), customizable with different
vegetables and fruits.

Harri's Sardine Sandwich with Mustard & Yogurt Butter

Ingredients:

- 2 cans sardines in oil, drained
- 4 slices of crusty bread
- 4 tablespoons plain yogurt
- 1 tablespoon Dijon mustard
- 1/2 teaspoon lemon juice
- 1/4 teaspoon fresh dill, chopped
- Salt and pepper to taste
- Optional: lettuce, tomato, and red onion slices for garnish

Nutritional Information (per serving):

- Calories: 300
- Fat: 15g (3g saturated)
- Carbs: 30g (2g fiber)
- Protein: 25g
- Calcium: 300mg (30% DV)

Cooking Time: 10 minutes

Serving Size: 4

Instructions:

1. Mash sardines with a fork in a bowl.
2. In a separate bowl, mix yogurt, Dijon mustard, lemon juice, and dill. Sprinkle some salt and pepper according to your taste preferences.
3. Spread the yogurt mixture onto the bread slices.
4. Top with mashed sardines and your favorite sandwich toppings (lettuce, tomato, red onion, etc.).
5. Enjoy a quick and nutritious protein-packed sandwich!

Label: Simple and tasty recipe, rich in calcium and omega-3 fatty acids, gluten-free option (use gluten-free bread), customizable with different spices and herbs.

Spinach and Ricotta Parcels

Ingredients:

- 12 wonton wrappers
- 15 ounces ricotta cheese
- 1/2 cup chopped spinach
- 1/4 cup grated Parmesan cheese
- 1/4 cup chopped fresh basil
- 1 egg yolk, beaten
- Olive oil for drizzling
- Salt and pepper to taste

Nutritional Information (per serving):

- Calories: 300
- Fat: 15g (5g saturated)
- Carbs: 25g (2g fiber)
- Protein: 20g
- Calcium: 300mg (30% DV)

Cooking Time: 20 minute

Serving Size: 4

Instructions:

1. Preheat the oven to 400°F (200°C). Line a baking sheet with parchment paper.
2. In a bowl, combine ricotta cheese, spinach, Parmesan cheese, basil, and salt and pepper to taste. Mix well.
3. Place a wonton wrapper on a flat surface. Brush the edges with beaten egg yolk.
4. Spoon a heaping tablespoon of ricotta mixture in the center of the wrapper.
5. Fold the wrapper diagonally into a triangle shape, pressing the edges to seal.
6. Repeat with remaining wonton wrappers and filling.
7. Brush the parcels with olive oil.
8. Put it in the oven for 15-20 minutes, or until it turns golden brown and crispy.
9. Enjoy warm as a light appetizer or main course.

Label: Versatile appetizer or light main course, rich in calcium and protein, vegetarian option, customizable with different fillings and herbs.

Pumpkin and Kale Soup

Ingredients:

- 2 tablespoons olive oil
- 1 onion, chopped
- 2 cloves garlic, minced
- 4 cups vegetable broth
- 2 cups chopped pumpkin flesh
- 2 cups chopped kale
- 1/2 cup heavy cream (optional)
- Salt and pepper to taste
- Pumpkin seeds and fresh herbs (optional) for garnish

Nutritional Information (per serving):

- Calories: 250
- Fat: 10g (2g saturated)
- Carbs: 30g (5g fiber)
- Protein: 5g
- Calcium: 200mg (20% DV)

Cooking Time: 30 minutes

Serving Size: 4

Instructions:

1. Warm up olive oil in a big pot on medium heat. Put in the onion and cook until it gets soft, around 5 minutes. Add garlic and cook for one more minute until it smells good. Pour in vegetable broth and bring it to a boil.
2. Add pumpkin and kale. Reduce heat and simmer for 20 minutes, or until pumpkin is tender.
3. Puree the soup with an immersion blender or in batches in a traditional blender until smooth.
4. Stir in heavy cream (optional) and season with salt and pepper to taste.
5. Serve hot, garnished with pumpkin seeds and fresh herbs (optional).

Label: Nutrient-packed and comforting soup, rich in vitamins and minerals, vegan option (omit cream), customizable with different spices and toppings.

Salmon and Broccoli Quiche

Ingredients:

- 1 (9-inch) frozen pie crust, thawed
- 1 tablespoon olive oil
- 1 onion, chopped
- 2 cloves garlic, minced
- 1 head broccoli, cut into florets
- 4 ounces smoked salmon, flaked
- 3 large eggs, beaten
- 1 cup milk
- 1/2 cup grated Gruyère cheese
- 1/4 teaspoon dried dill
- Salt and pepper to taste

Nutritional Information (per serving):

- Calories: 400
- Fat: 20g (5g saturated)
- Carbs: 25g (2g fiber)
- Protein: 30g
- Calcium: 250mg (25% DV)

Cooking Time: 45 minutes

Serving Size: 6

Instructions:

1. Warm olive oil in a pan on medium heat. Put in the onion and cook until it becomes soft, which should take about 5 minutes.
2. Add garlic and cook for another minute until fragrant.
3. Add broccoli florets and cook for 5-7 minutes, or until tender-crisp.
4. Spread the cooked broccoli and onion mixture evenly in the bottom of the pie crust.
5. Top with flaked salmon. Combine eggs, milk, Gruyère cheese, dill, salt, and pepper in a bowl. Whisk well until combined.
6. Pour the egg mixture over the salmon and broccoli filling, filling the crust nearly to the top. Bake for 35-40 minutes, or until the egg custard is set and the crust is golden brown. Check if a knife inserted into the middle comes out clean. Let the quiche cool for at

least 15 minutes before slicing and serving.
Enjoy warm or at room temperature.

Label: Delicious and satisfying main course, rich in calcium and protein, gluten-free option (use a gluten-free pie crust), customizable with different vegetables and cheeses.

Chicken and Vegetable Curry

Ingredients:

- 1 tablespoon olive oil
- 1 onion, chopped
- 2 cloves garlic, minced
- 1 inch ginger, grated
- 1 tablespoon curry powder
- 1 teaspoon ground turmeric
- 1/2 teaspoon cumin
- 1/4 teaspoon cayenne pepper (optional)
- 1 (14.5 oz) can of diced tomatoes, undrained
- 1 cup chicken broth
- One pound of boneless, skinless chicken thighs cut into small, bite-sized pieces.
- 2 cups chopped mixed vegetables (bell peppers, carrots, broccoli, etc.)
- 1 cup coconut milk
- 1/2 cup cooked brown rice, per serving
- Fresh cilantro and lime wedges for garnish (optional)

Nutritional Information (per serving):

- Calories: 400
- Fat: 15g (3g saturated)
- Carbs: 40g (5g fiber)
- Protein: 35g
- Calcium: 150mg (15% DV)

Cooking Time: 30 minutes

Serving Size: 6

Instructions:

1. Warm olive oil in a big pot or Dutch oven on medium heat. Put in the onion and cook until it gets soft approximately 5 minutes. Then, add garlic and ginger, and cook for one more minute until it smells good.
2. Stir in curry powder, turmeric, cumin, and cayenne pepper (optional). Cook for 1 minute, stirring constantly.
3. Add diced tomatoes, chicken broth, and chicken pieces. Bring to a simmer and cook for 10 minutes, or until chicken is cooked through.

4. Add chopped vegetables and coconut milk. Simmer for an additional 5-7 minutes, or until vegetables are tender-crisp.
5. Serve over cooked brown rice, garnished with fresh cilantro and lime wedges (optional).

Label: Flavorful and nutritious curry, a good source of protein and vitamins, customizable with different vegetables and spices, dairy-free option (use coconut milk or vegan yogurt).

Greek Salad

Ingredients:

- 4 cups mixed greens
- 1 cup chopped cucumber
- 1/2 cup chopped tomato
- 1/4 cup crumbled feta cheese
- 1/4 cup Kalamata olives, sliced
- 2 tablespoons red onion, thinly sliced
- 2 tablespoons olive oil
- 1 tablespoon lemon juice
- 1 teaspoon dried oregano
- Salt and pepper to taste

Nutritional Information (per serving):

- Calories: 300
- Fat: 15g (4g saturated)
- Carbs: 15g (3g fiber)
- Protein: 15g
- Calcium: 200mg (20% DV)

Cooking Time: 10 minutes

Serving Size: 2

Instructions:

1. In a large bowl, combine mixed greens, cucumber, tomato, feta cheese, olives, and red onion.
2. In a small jar, whisk together olive oil, lemon juice, oregano, salt, and pepper.
3. Drizzle the dressing over the salad and toss to coat.
4. Enjoy a refreshing and light salad packed with nutrients!

Label: Simple and flavorful salad, rich in calcium and antioxidants, vegan option (omit feta cheese), customizable with different ingredients and dressings.

Tofu and Vegetable Stir-Fry

Ingredients:

- 1 tablespoon vegetable oil
- 1 block (14 oz) extra-firm tofu, drained and pressed
- 1 cup chopped broccoli florets
- 1 cup chopped bell pepper (red or yellow)
- 1/2 cup chopped carrots
- 1/4 cup soy sauce
- 1 tablespoon rice vinegar
- 1 tablespoon honey
- 1 teaspoon toasted sesame oil
- 1/2 teaspoon grated ginger
- Cooked rice or noodles, for serving

Nutritional Information (per serving):

- Calories: 350
- Fat: 10g (1g saturated)
- Carbs: 40g (5g fiber)
- Protein: 25g
- Calcium: 100mg (10% DV)

Cooking Time: 20 minutes

Serving Size: 2

Instructions:

1. Warm oil in a big skillet or wok on medium-high heat. Cut tofu into cubes and put them in the pan.
2. Cook tofu for 5-7 minutes, or until lightly browned on all sides.
3. Add broccoli, bell pepper, and carrots. Cook by stirring for 5-7 minutes, or until the vegetables become tender.
4. In a small bowl, whisk together soy sauce, rice vinegar, honey, toasted sesame oil, and grated ginger. Pour the sauce over the vegetables and tofu in the wok.
5. Stir-fry for 1-2 minutes, or until the sauce is heated through and coats the ingredients.
6. Serve immediately over cooked rice or noodles. Enjoy a plant-based protein and vitamin-rich stir-fry!

Label: Hearty and filling vegetarian stir-fry, a good source of iron and fiber, gluten-free option (use gluten-free noodles), customizable with different vegetables and sauces.

Cheese and Tomato Pizza

Ingredients:

- 1 (12-inch) pre-made pizza crust
- 1/4 cup tomato sauce
- 1/2 cup shredded mozzarella cheese
- 1/4 cup chopped fresh basil leaves (optional)
- Olive oil and dried oregano for drizzle (optional)

Nutritional Information (per serving):

- Calories: 400
- Fat: 15g (5g saturated)
- Carbs: 40g (2g fiber)
- Protein: 20g
- Calcium: 300mg (30% DV)

Cooking Time: 15 minutes

Serving Size: 2

Instructions:

1. Preheat oven to 425°F (220°C). Line a baking sheet with parchment paper.
2. Spread tomato sauce evenly over the pizza crust.
3. Top with shredded mozzarella cheese.
4. Bake for 10-12 minutes, or until the crust is golden brown and the cheese is melted and bubbly.
5. Garnish with fresh basil leaves and a drizzle of olive oil and dried oregano (optional).
6. Enjoy a classic and simple homemade pizza!

Label: Comfort food made healthy, customizable with different toppings and cheeses, gluten-free option (use a gluten-free pizza crust), quick and easy recipe.

Conclusion

You have reached the end of this cookbook, but not the end of your journey. You have learned how to nourish your bones and your body, by following the recipes and tips in this book. You have also learned how to enjoy your food and your life, by discovering new flavors and cuisines. But there is always more to learn and more to explore. Some countless other foods and dishes can benefit your bone health and your overall well-being. There are endless ways to adapt and customize the recipes in this book to suit your tastes and needs. There are infinite possibilities to create your recipes and stories, using your creativity and passion. So don't stop here. Keep cooking, keep eating, keep living. Keep experimenting and trying new things. Keep taking care of yourself and your health. Keep inspiring and being inspired by others. And most importantly, keep smiling and keep shining. You are a star, and you deserve to sparkle. Thank you for choosing this cookbook. I hope you enjoyed it as much as I did. I hope you found it useful and helpful. I hope you will come back to it again and again. Until next time, bon appetit and happy cooking!

www.ingramcontent.com/pod-product-compliance
Lightning Source LLC
Chambersburg PA
CBHW060844260726
48661CB00002B/604